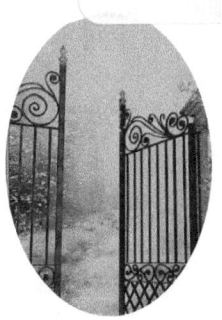

Pray Them to Heaven

Doris Gaines Rapp, Ph.D.

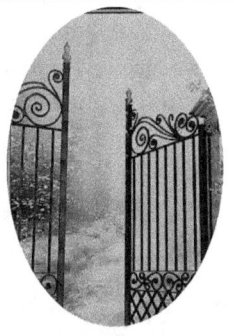

Pray Them to Heaven

Doris Gaines Rapp, Ph.D.

Huntington, Indiana

Copyright 2021 Doris Gaines Rapp

Daniel's House Publishing
Huntington, Indiana 46750

www.dorisgainesrapp.com
https://praythemtoheaven.blogspot.com
contact: dorisgainesrapp@gmail.com

All rights reserved. No part of this book may be used or reproduced in any form or by any electronic or mechanical means, including information storage and retrieval systems, without permission in writing from the author, except a reviewer who may quote brief passages in a review.

The Cover design is stock imagery from Dreamstime.com. Illustration 78301126
© Unholyvault | Dreamstime.com
Put in place by @Debi Lindhorst/The Type Galley.
Library of Congress Control Number: 2021906039

ISBN-13: 978-1-7365110-0-8 (paperback)
ISBN-13: 978-1-7365110-1-5 (eBook)

Table of Contents

Page	Chapter	
9	1	God Receives Them
18	2	Prayers for Others
32	3	Light Your Lamp
39	4	The Prayer We Know
46	5	The Lord's Prayer
56	6	A Prayer for the Non-believer
59	7	Family
66	8	Other Beliefs
76	9	The Visit
84	10	Life Can Move Fast
94	11	Grief Draws Near
102	12	He Laid it on My Heart

108	13	The Process
113	14	Pray them to Heaven
118		References
121		About the Author

Dedicated to all those who grieve.

Grieve no more.

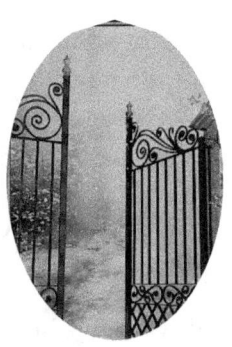

One

God Receives Them

Some ask why God takes people from their loved ones so soon. *I believe He takes no one but receives them when they arrive.*

Still, we feel helpless. We think we must be in control of everything, but we can't stop our friend or loved one from dying. So, it has to be someone's fault. And . . . we blame God.

We live in such divisive times we blame everyone else for everything else. Those *others* may be those of a different political party or philosophy, a different race, different religion, different sex, different . . .. You get the idea; they are "different."

Families have shunned family members who don't believe as they do. "I can't have them around. I don't agree with them."

As Christians, when those *others* are nearing death, some believers begin to panic. They fear they may not see their loved ones in Heaven because they didn't have the same beliefs here on earth.

Believing we have Heaven figured out, we grieve. Whether you're grieving over the death of someone you hold dear, you're a clergy member, counselor, hospice worker, or the always-ready-to-listen-friend people call when they're in pain, I'm sure many of you are familiar with the accusations people throw at God.

As a psychotherapist, I heard people blame God for everything in their lives that isn't perfect.

Who said the things of this world are supposed to be perfect? In Luke 18:19, Jesus said, "Why do you call me good? No one is good except God alone." And nowhere on earth is perfect. Only Heaven is perfect.

Some believe that God should be their genie-in-a-jug. All we should have to do is rub the magic bottle and God should grant our every wish. Instead, He sits up there in Heaven and waits until we're happy, then takes our loved one away from us. When grief hits, we have nowhere to turn.

A few months ago, I thought

there was nothing I could do when April, our daughter-in-law, was dying. She hadn't accepted Jesus, the son of God, as her Savior.

No—April followed the Pagan religion of Wicca, Pagan Witchcraft. So, I feared she would pass out of this world without knowing the wonderful love of our Savior, and the redemptive power of His saving grace. April was rapidly slipping away and I feared I wouldn't see her in Heaven.

To a Wiccan, the afterlife is in the Summerland. Wiccans believe they have many reincarnations. After their last incarnation, their highest level of an afterlife is Nirvana. As the Bible teaches us, these are not the beliefs leading to everlasting life in Heaven. That is why we don't believe we will see our loved ones on the other side. Their destination is not ours.

My friends, once we stand

before God, He is the one who decides and welcomes. It is God's Heaven and we all need to be in harmony with Him.

We have read that we must open the door to our heart ourselves for Christ to enter. The same is true of our entering into Heaven. We must decide to step through the entrance. I couldn't do it for her. Warner Sallman's beautiful painting of *Christ at Heart's Door* depicts that. Jesus stands outside the arched entry, knocking. There is no handle on the outside of the door. If He is going to be able to go in, we must be the ones to open the door to our hearts.

But what if someone we love can't even find the door or gate to the garden of Heaven; can we help them? Many may think I'm saying we can get someone "into" Heaven. No, as I said, salvation is an individual process. We must open the door. John 3:16 is clear. "For God so loved the world that he gave his one and only Son, that whoever believes in him shall not perish but have eternal life." (NIV)

While we cannot make a statement of faith about another's belief so they can enter into Heaven, or open the door for them, we can get someone "to" Heaven.

Then, I remembered a line from the Biblical passage in Acts 16: 24-34. A jailer had received orders to put Paul and Silas in prison.

> 24 When he [the jailer] received these orders, he put them [Paul and Silas] in the inner cell and fastened their feet in the stocks. 25 About midnight Paul and Silas were praying and singing hymns to God, and the other prisoners were listening to them.
>
> 26 Suddenly there was such a

violent earthquake that the foundations of the prison were shaken. At once all the prison doors flew open, and everyone's chains came loose.

27 The jailer woke up, and when he saw the prison doors open, he drew his sword and was about to kill himself because he thought the prisoners had escaped.

28 But Paul shouted, "Don't harm yourself! We are all here!"

29 The jailer called for the lights, rushed in, and fell trembling before Paul and Silas. 30 He then brought them out and asked, "Sirs, what must I do to be saved?"

31 They replied, "Believe in the Lord Jesus, and you will be saved—you and your household." 32 Then they spoke the word of the Lord to him and to all the others in his house. 33 At that hour of the night the jailer took

them and washed their wounds; then immediately he and all his household were baptized.

34 The jailer brought them into his house and set a meal before them; he was filled with joy because he had come to believe in God—he and his whole household. (NIV)

I thought of verse 31 again. "Believe in the Lord Jesus, and you will be saved—you and your household."

The jailer's belief in God did not save his family. His belief in God caused him to invite his family to come to know God for themselves and learn of His son, Jesus. Then, each member chose to believe. However, the jailer's faith did lead his family to Paul's teaching about God. In the broader sense, we call that evangelism.

When someone is in need, we want to do something, whatever that "something" is. When April became gravely ill, I got calls and messages from many friends and family who also felt helpless. They didn't know how to pray for someone when that someone didn't believe in the God to whom they prayed.

One asked, "Why does God always take the young ones? She is only forty-nine." Again . . . **I don't believe God takes anyone from their family and friends. I believe He receives them when they arrive home to Heaven.**

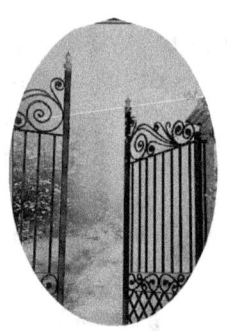

Two

Prayers for Others

Believers know the effectiveness of prayer. It has been a part of their experience and the experience of those they know for their whole lives as Christians.

Science has finally started to focus on prayer and research its power. The Spiritual Arts Institute reported on distance healing in an article, *Remote Healing Through*

Prayer, accessible on their blog.

Even Bahai teachings reported on the effectiveness of prayer for spiritual and physical healing, in an article published April 13, 2020. Their work, *Quantum Entanglement, Prayer and Healing*, explained the concept through an understanding of quantum physics and quantum entanglements. It is interesting and I encourage you to read the articles, but most Christians don't need research or proof of prayer. They live it.

I realize my use of the words, *pray someone to Heaven*, sounds different from what you're used to. And, we wonder, if the person is unconscious, how can they hear the prayer? If they are halfway around the world, we know they cannot hear our prayers with their physical ears.

Research shows that people thousands of miles away benefit from prayers offered on their behalf. Many of us pray daily for people on our prayer chain we don't even know.

Some may ask, "How can I pray them to Heaven? They already died. It's too late."

The Bible described some examples of believers who prayed for their loved ones' healing even after they died. Mark 5:22-42 described Jairus who came to Jesus as Jesus spoke to a crowd by the sea. This then is the testimony of Jairus, a synagogue leader, regarding his daughter.

> 22 Then one of the synagogue leaders, named Jairus, came, and when he saw Jesus, he fell at his feet.
>
> 23 He pleaded earnestly with him, "My little daughter is dying. Please, come and put your hands on her so that she will be healed

and live." 24 So Jesus went with him. [Notice, Jairus's daughter did not ask for healing; her father did.]

A large crowd followed and pressed around him. 25 And a woman was there who had been subject to bleeding for twelve years. 26 She had suffered a great deal under the care of many doctors and had spent all she had, yet instead of getting better, she grew worse. 27 when she heard about Jesus, she came up behind him in the crowd and touched his cloak, 28 because she thought, "If I touch his clothes, I will be healed." 29 Immediately her bleeding stopped and she felt in her body that she was freed from her suffering.

30 At once Jesus realized that power had gone out from him. He turned around in the crowd and asked, "Who touched my

clothes?"

31 "You see the people crowding against you," his disciples answered, "and yet you ask, "Who touched me?"

32 But Jesus kept looking around to see who had done it. 33 Then the woman, knowing what had happened to her, came and fell at his feet and, trembling with fear, told him the whole truth.
34 Daughter, your faith has healed you. Go in peace and be freed from your suffering."

35 While Jesus was still speaking, some people came from the house of Jairus, the synagogue leader. "Your daughter is dead," they said. "Why bother the teacher anymore?"

36 Overhearing what they said, Jesus told them, "Don't be afraid; just believe."
37 He did not let anyone follow him except Peter, James and

John the brother of James.

38 When they came to the home of a synagogue leader, Jesus saw a commotion, with people crying and wailing loudly. 39 He went and said to them, "Why all this commotion and wailing? The child is not dead but asleep.

40 But they laughed at him. After he put them out, he took the child's father and mother and the disciples who were with him and went in where the child was.

41 He took her by the hand and said to her," *Talitha koum!*" [which means "Little girl, I say to you, get up!"]

42 Immediately the girl stood up and began to walk around [she was twelve years old]. At this they were completely astonished. (NIV)

• • •

Most people know the story of

Lazarus. Jesus raised Lazarus four days after he died. In John 11:1-44 we find the testimony concerning Lazarus, the brother of Mary and Martha who lived in Bethany. When Lazarus became sick, his two sisters sent someone to bring Jesus so He could heal him.

> 1 Now a man named Lazarus was sick. He was from Bethany, the village of Mary, and her sister Martha. 2 [This Mary, whose brother Lazarus now lay sick, was the same one who poured perfume on the Lord and wiped his feet with her hair.] 3 So the sisters sent word to Jesus, "Lord, the one you love is sick."
>
> 4 When he heard this, Jesus said, "This sickness will not end in death. No, it is for God's Glory so that God's Son may be glorified through it." 5 Now Jesus loved Martha and her sister and Lazarus. 6 So when he heard that Lazarus was sick, he stayed

where he was two more days, 7 and then he said to his disciples, "Let this go back to Judea."

8 "But Rabbi," they said, "a short while ago the Jews there tried to stone you, and yet you're going back?"

9 Jesus answered, "Are there not twelve hours of daylight? Anyone who walks in the daytime will not stumble, for they see by this world's light. 10 It is when a person walks at night that they stumble, for they have no light."

11 After he had said this, he went on to tell them, "Our friend Lazarus has fallen asleep, but I am going there to wake him up."

12 His disciples replied, "Lord if he sleeps, he will get better."

13 Jesus had been speaking of his death, but his disciples thought he meant natural sleep.

14 So then he told them plainly,

"Lazarus is dead, 15 and for your sake, I am glad I was not there, so that you may believe. But let us go to him."

16 Then Thomas (also known as Didymus) said to the rest of the disciples, "Let us also go, that we may die with him."

17 On his arrival, Jesus found that Lazarus had already been in the tomb for four days.

18 Now Bethany was less than two miles from Jerusalem, 19 and many Jews had come to Martha and Mary to comfort them in the loss of their brother. 20 When Martha heard that Jesus was coming, she went out to meet him, but Mary stayed at home.

21 "Lord," Martha said to Jesus, "if you had been here, my brother would not have died. 22 But I know that even now God will give you whatever you ask." 23 Jesus said to her, "Your brother

will rise again."

24 Martha answered, "I know he will rise again in the resurrection at the last day."

25 Jesus said to her, "I am the resurrection and the life. The one who believes in me will live, even though they die; 26 and whoever lives by believing in me will never die. Do you believe this?"

27 "Yes, Lord," she replied, "I believe that you are the Messiah, the Son of God, who is to come into the world."

28 After she had said this, she went back and called her sister Mary aside. "The teacher is here," she said, "and is asking for you."

29 When Mary heard this, she got up quickly and went to him. 30 Now Jesus had not yet entered the village, but was still at the

place where Martha had met him. 31 When the Jews who had been with Mary in the house, comforting her, noticed how quickly she got up and went out, they followed her, supposing she was going to the tomb to mourn there.

32 When Mary reached the place where Jesus was and saw him, she fell at his feet and said, "Lord, if you had been here, my brother would not have died."

33 When Jesus saw her weeping, and the Jews who had come along with her also weeping, he was deeply moved in spirit and troubled.

34 "Where have you laid him?" he asked.

"Come and see, Lord?" they replied.

35 Jesus wept.

36 Then the Jews said, "see how

he loved him!"

37 But some of them and said, "Could not he who opened the eyes of the blind man have kept this man from dying?"

38 Jesus, once more deeply moved, came to the tomb. It was a cave with a stone laid across the entrance.

39 "Take away the stone," he said.

"But, Lord," Martha said, the sister of the dead man, "by this time there is a bad odor, for he has been there four days."

40 Then Jesus said, "Did I not tell you that if you believe, you will see the glory of God?"

41 So they took away the stone. Then Jesus looked up and said, "Father, I think you know that you have heard me. 42 I knew that you always hear me, but I

said this for the benefit of the people standing here, that they may believe that you sent me."

43 When he had said this, Jesus called in a loud voice, "Lazarus, come out!" 44 The dead man came out, his hands and feet wrapped with strips of linen and a cloth around his face.

Jesus said to them, "Take off the grave clothes and let him go." (NIV)

• • •

Jesus went to both homes because someone in the house believed He was Christ. Jairus, as well as Mary and Martha, knew Jesus had the power to ask God to heal their loved ones. Each was positive; they firmly believed Jesus could save the life of their daughter or brother.

In addition to our physical life, Jesus can save our spiritual life, our soul. He is both our savior and redeemer. He can save us *"from"* our sins [our savior] or save us *"in"* our sins [our redeemer]. As Redeemer Christ, He is willing to save us despite our sins.

Still, I worried and felt helpless. April was sick and her physician said her body was beyond repair. I couldn't see how she would find her way to Heaven when she didn't believe in God, and would not be able to recognize the voice of Jesus calling to her. Then, God told me, there was indeed something I could do.

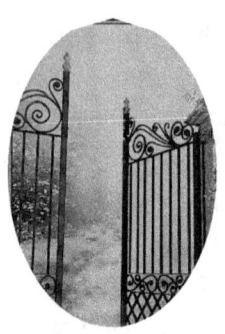

Three

Light Your Lamp

I would guide April, somehow, to Heaven. Like an old-world lamplighter, I knew I needed to trim my lamp and let my lower light send a gleam across April's path to guide her to the gate of Heaven. As the jailer, it was his faith in Jesus that shone the light for those in his household who didn't yet believe. The family had to choose on their own to follow the beam.

Praying for another can be our most important mission in life. Some older people feel useless. They feel it's past the time when they can make a difference in society. Praying for someone to make it home, is certainly not useless activity. Going home is everything in life. Those in retirement facilities have family and friends, like April in our family, who would benefit from their prayers. A prayer journal would be wonderful, so the journal keeper can go back weeks and months later to see the progress of their prayers.

Many years ago, an older lady brought her Prayer Journal to a women's meeting. As she turned the pages, she came to a section labeled, grandchildren.

"Now, they are my lovelies." She smiled as she softly patted the page. As she turned to previous entries, she was able to review past prayers and see, in writing, how the Lord had answered. Her prayers lit the way for others to find a blessing.

A favorite hymn often flows through my mind while I'm driving, or in the shower. The words ring true for me and summon me to join in.

You may remember the hymn, *Let the Lower Lights Be Burning* by Philip Bliss. If you can't call it to mind, your heart can. It may be a reminder of our responsibility to be a lower light, one of the lights along the shore, the light that gives a sailor, adrift on the sea, the light and hope to find their way home.

• • •

Let the Lower Light Be Burning
(Philip P. Bliss)

Brightly beams our Father's mercy,
From His Lighthouse evermore,
But to us, He gives the keeping
Of the lights along the shore.

> *Let the lower lights be burning!
> Send a gleam across the wave!
> Some poor fainting, struggling Seaman
> you may rescue, you may save.

Dark the night of sin has settled,
Loud the angry billows roar;
Eager eyes are watching, longing,
For the lights along the shore.

> *Let the lower lights be burning!
> Send a gleam across the wave!
> Some poor fainting, struggling Seaman
> you may rescue, you may save.

Trim your feeble lamp, my brother;
Some poor sailor, tempest-tossed,
Trying now to make the harbor,
In the darkness may be lost.
   *Let the lower lights be burning!
   Send a gleam across the wave!
   Some poor fainting, struggling Seaman
   you may rescue, you may save.

(Pub. 1871 – now in the public domain)

    God's lighthouse beams on everyone all of the time. Still, He tasks us with keeping the lower lights shinning, the ones running along the shore, guiding the stranded fisherman to a safe mooring.

    The job God gives us is not just a second thought, a little busywork, a non-important responsibility. The light we shine, will rescue a stranded traveler if we're a flame and not a hostile, dark presence. I had to shine my light along the shore in a way April could see.

Years ago, oil burned in the lamps that lit everyone's home. Ships at sea had crewmen to take care of the lamps on board. In the streets, some lamplighters lit each wick of the streetlights at sundown.

Part of the lamplighter's job was "trimming" the wick. The wick drew oil up from the reservoir at the bottom of the lamp. Trimming the wick allowed the flame to burn clean and bright. If the wick was poorly trimmed, the flame would be dim and smokey. Our wick needs to have the dead, burnt pieces cut away to make the flame from our lower light burn brighter. Remember to "trim" your wick, so you do not burn out too quickly, and the raggedness of the day does not dim your lamp.

I knew April would need a

clear, bright light to find her way home. I had to trim away doubt and narrow thinking. It was my job to be her lower light, because, "eager eyes are watching, longing, for the lights along the shore."

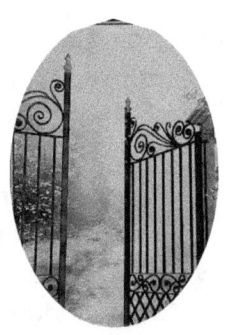

Four

The Prayer We Know

We, as Christians, are accustom to praying in the style and form Jesus taught His disciples. I'm certainly not changing the way Jesus taught us to pray. Jesus gave us a way to talk to God when the disciples asked Him to teach them how to pray. The Lord's Prayer provides the frame or outline for Prayer Therapy.

Roman Catholics pray The

Lord's Prayer, ending each time with ". . . deliver us from evil, Amen," each time they say the Rosary. Most Protestant churches pray the Lord's Prayer each Sunday Morning. The Lord's Prayer is often all that many people know of Prayer. Jesus taught us to pray and to intercede on someone's behalf, and that includes April and people who don't believe in the Lord or His prayer.

To understand the Lord's Prayer on a deeper level, I developed and taught Prayer Therapy while I was on the faculty of Tayler University in Upland, Indiana, long before I met April. The handouts I wrote provided a means to formalize and make the instructions consistent. Then, I expanded those handouts into a book, later titled *The Prayer Therapy of Jesus*.

Intercessory prayer falls in the

Prayer Therapy process within the area I call *Petition*, as you will note later on the chart. Petition is where we request something of God, that He give us our daily needs.

While creating the Prayer Therapy handouts, I developed the labels for each section of the Lord's Prayer so the one praying can put the prayer into their own words. It doesn't change what Jesus taught. It allows us to understand what we pray.

Petition is also where we pray for others in intercessory prayer, as well as lift up prayers for our healing, our need for encouragement, and the many other conversations with which we go to God. As parents, most of us pray often regarding our children. My prayers for April, during the years I knew her, included a petition that April recognize the God of Glory as He drew near to her. Praying April to Heaven came in the petition area of the prayer as well. However, the wording and approach were unique.

Christians pray. It is our opportunity to communicate with God. I know very little of how those of other faiths speak to their gods. I haven't studied the details of other religions and hadn't talked to April about it. Universities offer courses in comparative religions; however, I don't know if those syllabi include pagan religions.

At Christmas time a year or two ago, Bill, Katy, and I went over to the Dayton Mall to meet with Vonn, April, and the children. My sister, Donna, and brother-in-law Bob joined us at a wonderful pizza place near the shopping complex. Before we jumped into the pizza of my youth, with everything on it except anchovies,

I asked if it would be okay with everyone for Bill to say grace. From the side, I saw their youngest daughter, Saige, with wide eyes, glance quickly at her parents but said nothing. Vonn's simple answer was, "Sure." It appeared Vonn was still open to Christian prayer, or he knew how to be polite.

We have all prayed. My guess is, even those who don't believe in God, have argued with Him about His existence, therefore testifying to His presence. You can't argue with someone who isn't there.

One day Vonn called in a whisper, regarding a friend who was very sick. "Would you and Dad pray for him?" Vonn's voice was raspy and muffled. Not wanting April to hear him, he had taken his cell phone into the bedroom and spoke in hushed tones.

While I know very little about

Pagan beliefs, I have read, they pray at specific times using specific prayers. Their prayers are not to the Lord God, Jehovah. They direct their prayers to the Goddess and her companion. That is not a Christian's belief but Vonn needed for us to pray, to the father of our Lord Jesus Christ, on behalf of his friend. Also, April did welcome positive energy from others. We can always send love, or we are not followers of the author of love.

Some try to decide for God that a person cannot go to Heaven, because the one we pray for doesn't believe in Him. I thank God every day that I don't have to make any of His decisions. When we pray someone to Heaven, we don't withhold a blessing because we determine they don't deserve it. Our prayer is that our loved ones can find their way home. We experience deeper love and let go of the power we seek. We let God decide Godly things.

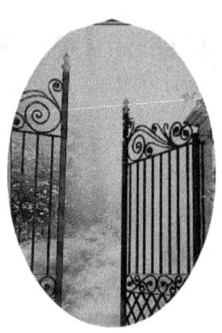

Five

The Lord's Prayer

I needed to pray for April, for her recovery, or for her to arrive at Heaven's gate. When God revealed the unique prayer to me, I understood God to mean, April was going home. The Prayer Therapy model is learning to pray specifically. A specific prayer follows the template as taught by our Lord. It includes a request that God releases us from specific negative emotions that rob us of our mental and physical health, energy, and well-being. In April's case, it would be a request for God to receive April when she arrives home, and that He will bless my attempt to guide her there.

Praying someone to Heaven is a specific element that fits into the Lord's Prayer. Pray intentionally, specifically, and watch the glory of God burst forth! God will answer those prayers specifically in His way.

Prayer Therapy is a form of prayer in which you pray selectively for release from the specific pain in your life that harms you, so God can answer specifically. When we pray someone to Heaven, we pray specifically that God will release them from the anger and pain that kept them trapped here on earth, and that they will see the Glory of God when they get to the garden of Heaven. The disciples asked Jesus to teach them how to pray and he gave them The Lord's Prayer.

On the following page, I have written the Lord's Prayer in segments or phrases, and have identified each segment's meaning. I know your immediate need is to pray for someone's healing or pray them to Heaven. At the risk of overpowering you with words that are too much for your current needs, I am listing the elements of the Lord's Prayer, so you have a clearer understanding of the prayer process with which most of us are familiar. The passage is from the New Testament book of Matthew.

• • •

Matthew 6: 9-12

King James Version

Acknowledgment:
    "Our Father, which art in Heaven,"
Reverence/Worship:
    Hallowed be thy name.
Pray for Christ's return:
    Thy kingdom come,
Surrender:
    thy will be done on earth as it is in Heaven.
Petition:
    Give us this day our daily bread.
Prayer for forgiveness:
    And forgive us our debts as we forgive our debtors.
Deliverance from our sins:
    And lead us not into temptation but deliver us from evil.
Acknowledge His Omnipresence:
    For thine is the kingdom,
Acknowledge His Omnipotence:
    and the power,

Relinquishing credit to God:
    and the glory, forever.
Closing:
    Amen."
*Claiming Christ's Power:

    In the name of Jesus Christ, or
        by the power of Jesus Christ.
*Prayer Therapy
    A specific, personal petition.
*Intercession
    Specific prayers for others.

*Identifies items not mentioned in Matthew 6.

*Secret Prayer

• • •

Once we have learned to pray, we can begin a new life, using what I call, the Secret Prayer. The secret prayer is a prayer for anonymous service. Each morning I ask God to use me in someone's life, that I may say something or do something on their behalf, so their life may be better, and they may be nearer to Him. But I do not want to know when it happened, or with whom it happened, so that I may not boast. All glory must go to God. It is a wonderful adventure.

Jesus told the disciples not to pray to draw attention to themself. We are to pray, focusing on God, and not on who may see us or admire our lofty words.

We identified the phrases of the Lord's Prayer, on the previous pages, so we can put each line into our own words.

Prayer Therapy falls within the fifth segment of the prayer, labeled "Petition," the section where we pray for specific needs. "Needs" can be "daily bread" or freedom from anger, jealously, or other negative emotions. Prayer is the portal to the divine. Don't be afraid to step through.

In Parker and St. John's book, *Prayer Can Change Your Life*, they described their scientific study involving the effectiveness of prayer over sixty years ago. In the nine-month study, medical tests gave beginning measurements, like X-rays, MRIs, and other relevant tests. Physicians compared that initial data with the test results at the end of the study. Most of the participants improved their health by a method of specific praying: naming negative emotions they prayed God to rid them of, and not just random praying.

Negative emotions make us weak and, over time, can make us sick. I am not saying, "It's all in your head." But, if your head isn't in the game of health, your score will fall like a concrete basketball.

Some agreed to pray, saying they pray every day, but wouldn't use prayer therapy. With fixed jaws, they announced, "I don't need to be taught how to pray."

Random, non-specific prayers, did not affect any improvement in their health. A random prayer would be the type we whisper as we run out the door in the morning.

- "Help me to do well on the test today."

- "Help me to get along with my boss."

- "Let this day be better than yesterday."

A specific prayer includes a request that God releases us from specific negative emotions which rob us of our mental and physical health, energy, and wellbeing. "For today, Father God, release me from the jealousy I feel toward my co-worker, Jane."

I am not suggesting you attempt to "cure" your physical, emotional, or family problems without professional help. Prayer Therapy can accompany proper psychological and medical treatment if needed, or stand-alone.

In my own life, physical healing occurred when others prayed with me for improvement in medical test results. In my private practice, I have witnessed patients' emotional health improve, as well as their relationships with others, through praying for specific needs, a "release of the captives." Then, go about the rest of the day, knowing God heard your prayer.

When we petition God, it's a form of prayer called supplication. My supplication to God was, that He would release April from whatever anger she may hold, search April's soul, and find anything in her that He could recognize as a child of His. With all of the love she had for her family, I knew He would. She was *family* and we lead *family* to God.

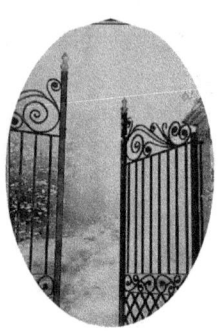

Six

A Prayer for the Non-Believer

As a parent, naturally, I pray for all my children. Even long before April became ill, my prayers went to God on her behalf.

Some admit they pray for their non-believing family members. But they don't believe God will welcome them into Heaven because of their non-belief. Some have taken more extreme measures. They have discontinued contact with them.

Since April was a non-believer, I didn't know if those of the Pagan religion pray, but like the jailer in the Bible's account of Paul and Silas, that didn't change my need to pray for her. The following prayer is like the prayers I sent to the Lord on Vonn and April's behalf. If you have a loved one or friend who is a non-believer, you may want to modify the prayer to meet your family's needs.

> "Holy Father of Jesus our Lord, and author of Love, I bow before your precious name. May your kingdom come swiftly so that your will is complete in my life and the lives of our children, just as the angels in Heaven now experience. For today, I ask that you pour out your glory on our son, Vonn, and his wife, April. Fill them so full of the

warmth of your love, they cannot fail to know it is you who touches them. Bless their lives so that they may bless others with your light. Rid their lives of negative emotions that they may enjoy good health. Where there is disappointment, please plant hope. Where there is anger, instill peace and love. Forgive me when I may not have demonstrated your presence in my life but have boasted of my relationship with you. It is only through Jesus, my redeemer, that I can claim your blessing, not through anything I may have done on my own. For to you belong all glory and honor. In the name of, and by the power of your son Jesus, the Christ, I pray. Amen."

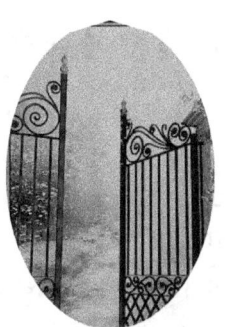

Seven

Family

Family is the place where you receive love, even when philosophies and ideas differ. Vonn switched to the Pagan religion too when he married April.

Years ago, we adopted Vonn when he was nearly ten years old. He joined our family of two daughters and another son.

The adoption agency told us, while his birth father was at work, his birth mother took him, his brother and sister, to a local orphanage and said, "Here, you take them. I don't want them anymore."

Social Services split up the three children into different homes. His birth father was unable to get them back.

Placed first with a farm family, Vonn's foster father got so frustrated with him one day, he threw him in a filthy pen with the pigs.

Vonn's next foster placement was with a woman who loved him very much. However, when she took Vonn's side in an issue at school, Social Services removed him from her home.

His last placement was in an experimental home, with a Jewish family. It was Vonn's privilege to recite the prayer after the lighting of the Friday night candles, before the Sabbat meal.

Baruch ata Adonai, Eloheinu Melech ha-olam, asher kidshanu b'mitzvotav vitzivanu l'hadlik ner shel Shabbat.

It means: Blessed are You, God, Ruler of the universe, who sanctified us with the commandment of lighting Shabbat candles. After we adopted Vonn, when it was his turn to offer grace at mealtime, we asked him to recite the Shabbat prayer so he would not forget it.

In our home, Vonn went with us to our Christian church every Sunday from the time the agency placed him there until he was out on his own. Yet, he was always looking for the bazaar, the unique.

Although Attention-Deficit/

Hyperactive-Disorder, Dyspraxia [now called Developmental coordination disorder], and a fascination with a fantasy life were some of the issues with which Vonn struggled, he grew a lot in our home. At first, he had trouble recognizing facial expressions or even understanding their meaning. As time went on, he developed a real sense of humor.

As a young adult, he married and had two daughters, Kathleen and Amanda. Neither he nor their mother was able to parent them at that time. When Katy was a few days old, Child Protective Services removed her from their home. Placed in a temporary foster home, the family loved and cared for her.

After hiring an attorney, Bill and I brought her home. We decided to rear her as our own. Leenie, Katy's nickname until high school, was six weeks old when we drove her from Ohio to our home in Muncie, Indiana. We officially adopted her at the end of the first year.

Amanda was born when Katy was thirteen months old. Her birth mother took Mandi to Texas, fearing she would lose her as well. Texas authorities called me at my office at Taylor University and told me they placed Amanda in a temporary foster home. Would I come out and testify that we had adopted her sister? I flew to Dallas and brought Mandi back to Indiana with me. She was seven months old and Katy was twenty months. With a grandson who was three years old, we started parenting a second family.

One day, Katy asked, "When baby go home?"

I smiled. "Baby is home,

Sweetie. She isn't going anywhere."

Eventually, Vonn and his first wife divorced. He floundered until he met April several years later. She became a stabilizing presence in his life.

Earlier, before she met Vonn, April worked at a daycare center. She was a gifted childcare worker. When the parents of one of the children under her care went back to England, they invited April to go along to enjoy some vacation time. Their generosity also extended to Vonn. Touring in London was a wonderful experience for both of them. Vonn became a hard and steady worker, a good husband and father to the three children born to them.

Vonn worked hard and April took care of the family details. Vonn said recently, "April was the organized one." Vonn brought in the income. They made a good couple.

April was great at finding bargains. With a limited income, she was able to find the things the children wanted by clipping coupons and searching the overloaded tables at yard sales. Still, there were a few major issues on which we didn't agree.

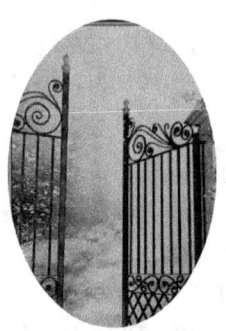

Eight

Other Beliefs

April and I didn't share the same religion or the same God. As I said, April followed the pagan religion. She was a Wiccan.

• • •

Wicca is a form of modern paganism, founded in England during the mid-twentieth century. Believers claim it is much older and originated before the

Christian religion. Wicca is another term for Pagan Witchcraft, a modern pagan religion. Scholars say it is both a new religious movement and is part of the occultist stream of Western esotericism.

Many adherents to Wicca use the pentacle [a disc-shape with a pentagram on top of it] and place it on a Wiccan altar to honor the elements of Earth, wind, fire, water, spirit, and the directions. The Earth element is in the north, air in the east, fire in the south, and water in the west.

Pagan religions today, hold several world views: pantheistic (a belief that all forces in the universe are God, but God doesn't have an individual personality), polytheistic (a belief in more than one god), animistic (a belief that everything - words, objects, places, nature, and creatures have a distinct spiritual essence), or monotheistic (a belief in one god).

I'm not a scholar of Paganism or Wiccan beliefs. Like others who search for ideas outside of their knowledge, I found information on Paganism and Wicca on Wikipedia on the internet. I'm also not teaching you about the topics. Since these are not my beliefs, I would not attempt to explain them in any deep sense of understanding. I would be a poor educator of a religion in which I do not believe nor have faith in any of its teachings.

I am merely explaining how it is possible to love a family member who holds opposite beliefs, because the God in whom I believe and worship, is the God of all, the God of Love. Love them for who they are that is loving.

Vonn and April were together for several years before they married. The wedding didn't take place in a little chapel or holy sanctuary. It was within a roped-off circle in their yard with a Pagan or Wiccan minister officiating in a black robe and Tabard, or open-sided tunic over it. Those not of the Pagan faith sat on chairs outside the circle, where they could observe.

Did we feel excluded? Of course not. Our inclusion was with those outside the circle, who believe in the Lord God, Jehovah, or at the very least, do not believe in Pagan Gods and Goddesses. We were there to show our love for our son and his new wife.

Christians often attend the many dances of Native Americans. Some dances are often part of religious rituals and ceremonies. Other dances, performed around a campfire, were to guarantee successful hunts and harvest, and for giving thanks to Wakan Tanka, the Great Spirit. But they won't go to their own child's wedding, celebrated in a church of a different denomination or faith.

Missionaries in Hawaii, Africa, and other places, attended local activities to honor the people, not to worship their foreign gods. King Kamehameha II of Hawaii, abolished some religious dining practices and instilled the luau in 1819. And, we all know of the many Pagan beliefs and activities attached to the celebration of Halloween. Does that mean we are Pagan? Of course not. We may dress up like a rabbit but we don't believe we're part of the rodent family.

Our main purpose should be to honor and support our children or family member. When we bring the love of Christ with us, we worship only

God and His son, Jesus. Maintaining contact is the only way to show them your God through the way you live.

Due to the distance between our homes, we didn't get to see the family very often. It's different from stopping in on the way home from work or bringing the children over when the neighbors on our street deck out their homes for beggars' night. Our time together became brief comments on social media, telephone calls, and the occasional visit. The year-of-the-pandemic, 2020, pre-vented face-to-face contact.

In October, despite Covid-19, we felt blessed that we were able to go to Ohio and see the house Vonn and April purchased, and moved into just months before.

April and Vonn had always rented. They never had a home of their own. She called me in the latter part of 2019. Their landlord had asked them to move as she was needing to move back into her country home. It caught Vonn and April off guard as April didn't remember their friend talking about moving back into her house so soon.

The issue wasn't just a home for the two of them and their three children. By that time in the life of their family, they had added three dogs, and a potbellied pig or two. Since they were renters, April was worried about finding a rental home where animals were welcome. A little poodle may have been acceptable, but their traveling menagerie was another thing.

The children enjoyed homeschooling long before the pandemic made distance learning an experience for many. So, finding a home in a particular school district was not necessary. Serenity was about fourteen years old at the time, Ray thirteen, and Saige was eleven, so space was of greater importance. It is one thing to have three toddlers running around the house, but quite another to find a home large enough for three nearly grown young people and all their trappings.

April was busy with the children's home-schooling, so I went online and looked for rental properties in southern Ohio. When I sent a picture and description of a house, April wasn't sure of what I found. It was a home for sale, on several acres, with some out-buildings for the animals.

"It isn't that we have bad credit, Mom." April's voice was a jumble of reality and the thrill of finding a forever home. The house and property met all their needs. And, it ticked off many of their wish-list items as well. "It's that we have no credit at all," she explained. "We pay cash for everything."

"I understand." Truly, I did. Stepping into homeownership can seem like a luxury unavailable to everyone. I certainly didn't want to push them. They were far more aware of their financial situation than I. "But if you think you can, you may want to do the math and check into the house I found. Sometimes, mortgage payments are lower than rent. I know of someone who bought their first house recently. While the process required a lot of paperwork and a bulldog's ability to hang on to every detail, they got their home."

April and Vonn began climbing the mountain of paperwork involved with a mortgage application and hopeful homeownership after their first tour of the country place.

As I remember it, the closing for the mortgage came after the first of the year, 2020, before COVID-19 kept everyone inside. After that, no one left their home or traveled for many months. Shelter-in-place orders kept people around the world inside. By the spring of 2020, half of the world's population was under a lockdown order. It wasn't until October, when there was a slight stabilization in the spread of the virus, that Bill, our daughter Kathleen (Katy), and I went to Ohio to see Vonn and April and the girls, and the first home of their own.

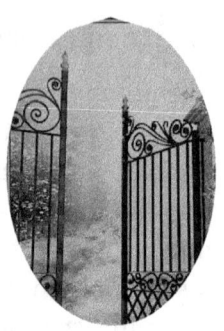

Nine

The Visit

It was late autumn, and the foliage along the roads through Indiana and Ohio was ablaze with the magnificent colors of fall when God loads His largest paintbrush with amber and gold to decorate His world. It looked like He hung lanterns in the forest to celebrate the end of the harvest.

We had no idea how fast life would change after our visit with

Vonn and April. We had worked through the differences between our families and chose not to argue about them. All an argument does is make the other person's position stronger. That enjoyable visit was only a short time before April's illness worsened.

During my psychology practice, I worked with some parents and their adult children who became estranged, due to differences in their beliefs and/or lifestyle. These are families in which at least one member says, "I can't have them in my life. They're against what I believe. I just can't talk to them anymore."

As I said, April's religious beliefs were vastly different from ours. However, her desire to parent her children was like all mothers. Vonn and April didn't have a lot of extra money, but that was alright. The family was her life. Even her social media description listed, "Wife, Mom, Cook, Referee, Boo-Boo Fixer, etc. as April is a stay-at-home mom."

I didn't agree with the way she handled kids' chores. She constantly expressed negative expectations, a form of reverse psychology. "I want them to clean the kitchen, but I know they won't." That becomes a self-fulfilling prophecy. They do not do what you expected them not to do.

Since April became ill, the thought came to me, perhaps her negative chore instructions reflected the pain she was in. Pain can drain one of energy and the strength to complete a task. At a minimum, it can raise blood pressure. Perhaps she couldn't parent in a positive tone, any more than the kids could complete their chores with a positive, work-well-done approach.

In parenting, I believe that a task should be set, and then the parent should expect the children to complete the job. Arguing as to which approach is better does nothing to change a parenting plan. It only broadens the void between families. Honestly, April didn't argue about any suggestions I made. As she grew sicker, she just sounded so helpless and deplete of the energy necessary to follow through.

Remember, you may not have all the answers as to why your adult children have chosen an opposite philosophy of life. It is then, that love forms a link on which to bridge the gap. Back and forth across the golden threads, a family can safely traverse. We must continue the dialog, to find all the other areas of life in which mutual understanding is present. You can never influence another if you aren't talking to them.

Due to the two-hundred-mile distance, we hadn't gotten as close to Serenity, Ray, and Saige as I would have liked. Vonn and April had only come to Indiana a few times. I had several major surgeries and a fall that resulted in a broken wrist. It had been very difficult for us to get to southern Ohio as well.

When we tried to talk on the cell phone, April always put it on speaker. That made our telephone conversations scattered and hard. One child would buzz into sound range after the other, usually not identifying which one they were. Sometimes, a lot of dead air made it uncertain if the family had gone into town for ice cream cones and forgot to end the call. However, in the larger picture of love for family, it didn't matter how often we'd spent quality face-time. It mattered that we cared about each other.

Serenity is a gifted hairstylist already, although only in her middle teens. At this point in her life, she hopes to go to cosmetology school. She can braid hair into beautiful styles, a skill I could never accomplish.

Ray was quiet when we last saw them and sadness seemed to overshadow the few smiles. Perhaps worry about April's health, even before the physician's appointment, was a reason. Ray enjoys writing and may work on two or three books at the same time. Writers are sometimes quiet. I haven't read any of her writing yet. One day perhaps Ray will let me enjoy all her creative thoughts she puts on paper.

Saige is very outgoing. She was proud to read me a story she'd written. She is bright and excited about life. Perhaps we'll have several Rapp authors in the family.

The children were thrilled to show us their new home and the out-buildings, where Rosie, their pot-bellied pig lived. To the left of the pig enclosure, a chicken coup housed many, hand-held chickens of several breeds. Saige carried the hens around within the wired off yard like they were small kittens. A wildflower field was between the yard and the back property line.

Regardless of our important differences, these things I know; the God of mercy, creation, and salvation, loved April and her family. He made her. He knew her.

While April didn't believe in the one God who created the Universe, and all that is in it, that didn't stop my prayers on her behalf. I prayed because I believe, not because April believed.

As I tell you about these few

days of April's passing over, you may find my words are synonyms for expressions you heard in the past. Some of you will reject what I am writing because I chose to use a broader vocabulary. My experience with prayer may be a little different from yours. That's alright. I only ask you to listen to what happened.

This rather small book is my testimony of the events that unfolded in April's last few days, not my effort to add additional lines to scripture. The Bible completed many years ago, needs no words of mine. Once a pen wrote the final word, nothing else needed saying. I'm not expanding the Bible or even interpreting it. I am bearing witness to what God laid on my heart.

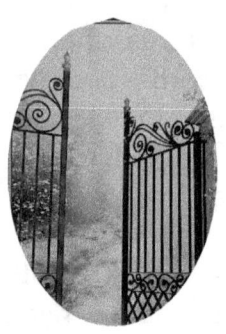

Ten

Life Can Move Fast

We didn't know how sick April was when the blue sky over their home was full of blowing leaves from the wooded area beyond the backfield. That was October 10, less than three months ago. At that time, April told us then that she hadn't been feeling well. She had been seeing her general practitioner for several months who put her on a round of antibiotics.

When that didn't cure her bladder infection, he switched to a different antibiotic. Still, the symptoms persisted. On October 12, the Monday following our visit, she had a medical appointment for a further test, a CT scan of her bladder. She was glad she was finally going to get some answers. April always wanted to get to the source of a problem.

After she kept her appointments for tests and consultation, April and Vonn called on speakerphone. She had a blood clot in her bladder and something appeared in the corner of her lung. Also, her blood count was very low. Later that day, Vonn posted a message on social media; April needed a blood transfusion. While at the emergency room, the medical team flushed out the bladder, and gave her an antibiotic through her I.V. The following day, along with an order for more blood work, the physician delivered some devastating news. The blood clot that appeared on the CT, was not. It was a tumor in her bladder. By 4:30 PM that day, she had her third bag of blood. October 14 began with an additional bag of blood before they began a procedure, a scope to determine the problems in the bladder.

October 15 opened with the possibility of going home later that day. April's physician came in at 7:35 AM and reported that her blood count had stabilized. She would need to come back the following Monday to get the pathology results from the scope. But the doctor said he was sure it was bladder cancer.

On the sixteenth, following the scope procedure, April called from her hospital room. She said the doctor reported cancer had gotten into her bladder wall or muscle. She was still reeling from her surgeon's brief after-surgery visit. April had very few answers at that point, except the news of a large presence of cancer. In a daze, she said the doctor delivered the news of her diagnosis, "apologized and left the room." She didn't know what he was sorry about. The nurse who followed him into April's room gave a few more details.

I saw no need to upset her further. I believed the doctor was not apologizing for anything he did. He was sorry there was little he could do but hope to save her life. Since cancer had gone through her bladder wall, some options were off the table. He referred her to Ohio State University. My husband and I, our extended family, our church family, and all of April's many friends and family prayed for healing and a positive, uplifting attitude.

April spent the next few days

getting a hospital bag packed so she would be ready when OSU called. On November 11, she went to Columbus to see the surgeon. He discussed the surgery and set up appointments with other physicians involved with the surgery and after-care.

On November 19 she went back to Columbus for another CT of the bladder and consultations with her anesthesiologist and plastic surgeon, and more bags of blood.

After returning home that day, she received a call from OSU. The medical team saw a blood clot in the vein that goes to her kidney. She needed to return to Columbus the next day for an Ultrasound. A half-hour later, the surgeon called and said he decided to not do the ultra-sound but would admit her to the hospital the next day. Twenty-five minutes after that, OSU called again and wanted her to come into the hospital that night. By 9:30 PM, they settled her into her room at the James Cancer Center at Ohio State. At 11:30 PM the doctor came in for a discussion of her blood.

Fast, so fast, everything moved like a great wind in a forest fire. At 8 AM November 20, a nurse hooked up another pint of blood, and at 11:35 April was already on the second bag, along with a discussion of a blood thinner. Later that day, the team did an Ultrasound of her legs and a CT scan of her chest.

By 6 AM, on November 21, many physicians were in and out of her room. Plans and more plans, faster and faster. The next day she had two more units of blood.

At 6:50 AM, on November 23, she talked to her doctor about the MRI for the blood clot in the vein so they would know how to plan during the surgery. April listened carefully but her heart was yearning to go home for Thanksgiving. At 11:45 AM the kidney specialist came in. She reported they wouldn't do the MRI since she could see all she needed to see on the previous images.

The surgery was only one week away. April began another unit of blood before going home.

On November 24, April was back home, thanks to a friend who drove to Columbus to pick her up. Before checking out, April talked to the doctor who said they would re-admit her on Sunday after Thanksgiving.

At home, there was so much to do. Besides Preparations for Thanksgiving and the Christmas decorations needed to go up. The children were a great help. April knew she wouldn't feel like supervising them after her surgery. So, the tree stood tall in the front window on November 25 and the Thanksgiving baking began. They filled the pantry the day after Thanksgiving. Together, they prepared the house and kitchen for her time in the hospital.

On Sunday, November 29, at 11:25 AM, April went back to OSU. Vonn had to work, so a friend drove her to Columbus. On November 30, at 5:40 AM, April was awake and feeling nervous. The nurse gave her another pint of blood, in preparation for surgery later that day.

April knew going into the procedure, if they removed the bladder, she would wear an ostomy bag the rest of her life. So, that was no surprise. The bag was a life-saving necessity. During the surgery, the surgeon put the stoma, or connection for the exterior urine bag, into place.

Things looked promising. April slept after surgery.

On December 1, doctors came in to check the incision. By 9:30 AM, a physical therapist had her up and out of bed to sit in a chair. April even took a few steps and a little walk. The next day, December 3, regular food was on her tray. She hadn't slept much during that night, so a nurse helped her take a walk around the floor at 4 AM. The blood clot was still there but the medical team expected it to dissolve. The best part, the team began to talk about her going home.

That night, April was thrilled to be home but had to sit up in the living room chair to sleep. At 12:30 PM the Home Health Care "lady" came.

Then, things happened. On December 7, her drain lines began leaking. They came completely out the next day. On December 9, she posted on Facebook that her abdominal muscles across the front of her stomach were tightening. One time, they all tightened at once, which caused her to double over.

On November 30, a surgeon tried to rescue her from the ravages cancer inflicted. The surgery to intervene in her bladder cancer was successful. Yes, her life would have forever changed, but she would have lived to love and nurture her husband and three children. Things didn't turn out that way.

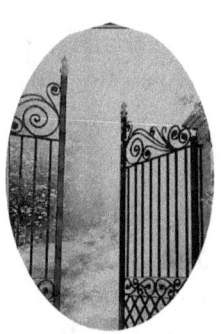

Eleven

Grief Draws Near

After April's surgery and her return home, she Messaged me. We typed back and forth for a while, then she called when she needed more talk time. She was concerned she may have come home from the hospital too early to celebrate their first holiday season in their new home.

    Her voice was strong but concerned. "I'm upset. Vonn thinks I manipulated the doctor into letting me come home. I didn't. The doctor said they wouldn't do an MRI on the weekend. So, I could go home, and then come back."

"I know," I empathized with her. And I did know. I knew our son, Vonn. People have an innate need to make everything right, to repair the broken shovel, put a Band-Aid on a fresh cut, and protect the family. "Vonn is worried and feels helpless. There's nothing he can do."

Encouraged by her positive attitude, I let her know how proud I was of her. She fully expected to adjust to her new way of living and being. She was sure she would handle wearing the exterior bladder pouch and live to take care of her family.

April had a follow-up visit with the surgeon the following week. It was after that medical appointment in

Columbus, as Vonn started to drive April back home, that the reason for her recent days of stomach muscle soreness became evident. When she started throwing up, Vonn turned the minivan around and took her back to the hospital.

She admitted she couldn't keep down the anti-blood-clotting medication the doctor prescribed, so she stopped taking it. When a clot cut off life-giving nourishment to her intestines, the damage was more than her body was able to repair and heal.

Our daughter-in-law, April, was dying of complications following a successful bladder cancer surgery. Her physician moved her to the hospital's hospice unit and kept her in a comfort state. That meant, the medical staff would give her pain medication and anti-anxiety meds, but when her blood pressure dropped or her heart stopped, they would allow her to pass on peacefully.

The blood clot changed it all. Nine weeks after we sat around the table at the Ponderosa in October in southern Ohio, the blood clot cut off life to April's lower digestive system. Her intestines died, as well as the stoma. Another surgery was not possible.

• • •

Again, prayers went up for a miracle. When miraculous healing did not take place, there was nothing anyone could do. But God laid on my heart, "That's not all."

God placed on my understanding one final blessing. While I waited, I learned Do not grieve what God wanted to reveal to me . . . a prayer to lead April to Heaven.

I know there will be some who

will argue with me about these things. They may say, "But that isn't Biblical." I cannot decide for God what His blessings may be. You're right, and neither can you. All I know is, these are the things He placed on my heart.

I know I can't save someone else. Their salvation is not mine to work out. Each person must decide and ask the Christ Jesus to come into their life. We are merely there to direct them along their way.

• • •

Late in the evening on December 10, the hospital called and asked Vonn to drive back to Columbus, Ohio. They didn't expect April to live through the night and wanted him to be able to say goodbye. They said he couldn't bring the children due to the COVID-19 epidemic. They barred visitors of any age from the hospital.

"If the kids can't come, then I won't be there either." Vonn was firm. "My kids are losing their mother. I won't leave them here alone. They need to see her one last time, too."

He simply could not drive two hours up to Columbus and two hours back while the children paced the floor, alone and afraid, back a long dark lane at home.

At first, the hospital personnel didn't seem to want to understand. Finally, after some discussion and Vonn's persistence, they permitted him to bring the children for one last goodbye.

The darkness of the night at 10 PM added to the gloom they all felt as they drove north along I-71. The oncoming headlights cast eerie shadows inside the minivan, lighting faces that remained dark with grief.

Inside the hospital, the long

corridors were empty except for people hurrying past in various colors of scrubs. If the hospital permitted visitors, smiling, and talking to family and friends, they would have all wandered home for the night by that time. But no one went in and out of the rooms. The clicking of shoes was all the family heard as they walked to room 720.

April's doctor ordered a medication that would bring her out of the medically induced coma so she would know they were there. As the children leaned close, April whispered something to each of the children. Vonn said her voice was weak so he couldn't hear what she told each one. One by one, the kids kissed their mother goodbye.

They only had a few minutes. There was no sitting in the waiting room or pacing the halls just to be close by. They had to drive back home, leaving April to slip slowly away alone.

So, Vonn and the children went home and . . . waited.

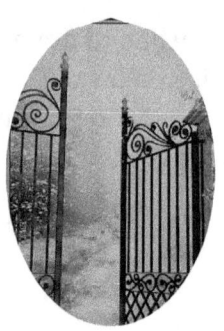

Twelve

He Laid it on My Heart

God gave me a full plan, right there on that Sunday morning, when I felt so helpless. "What can I do?" I cried out silently to God.

I finally surrendered. "I can do nothing," I whispered inside. "How do I pray for a non-believer? She doesn't believe in you, God, or your power to heal."

Thoughts kept swirling in my

head. My mind was on April and the whole family. They were all hurting. A torrent of prayers flooded over me. It was 9 AM, on December 13, 2020.

As I sat there in the church, the Lord began to give me answers to the questions I just hadn't been able to figure out on my own. His words came to me in beautiful snatches and images.

This was my experience, and I pass it on to you. It is what the Lord gave to me. I am a psychologist and novelist. Although my husband is a pastor, and I am not, I'm often called on to minister to church people outside of my private practice.

When grief hits, expectedly or unexpectedly, many people need to talk to someone about the emotional pain they are in. What I know is, God laid these thoughts on my heart and tasked me with obeying

His voice and testifying to these events.

That morning's service was full of the magical songs of Christmas. They filled my heart with love and light. As the music played and the congregation sang, I couldn't take my mind off April.

The lyrics told the story of how the son of God came to earth to usher in the dawning of forgiveness between people, and love for all. My heart warmed with His presence. I quickly fumbled in my purse for a pen, grabbed the back of my church bulletin, and wrote as fast as I could. While April lay in a hospital nearly one hundred seventy miles away, in a coma, I followed God's lead and prayed His prayer for her.

Off and on, for the rest of the day, I prayed that unique prayer. During the afternoon and evening, I entered and expanded my notes into my computer, and paused often to pray for April using the prayer God gave me.

That special sequence of prayer is what God laid on my heart that morning. Every time I prayed, I felt Him close to me. God gave me this understanding. "After you've finally acknowledged there is nothing else you can do . . . then do this."

When someone we love nears their time of home-going, I know we grieve. That is a perfectly natural reaction to loss. While I know grief will pass and memories will replace sorrow, that doesn't mean we will feel no pain as we walk through the valley of despair. Sometimes we feel angry, or guilty over our inability to stop our loved one's passing. We may also experience anxiety, sadness, and even despair.

We are "doers." We all seek something we can do to solve most problems, like the death of someone we know. We grieve over the dear one who is passing; and, we grieve over our inability to "do something" to prevent the loss.

The doctors told our son, "There's nothing anyone can do."

Christian friends contacted me, expressing their grief over April's illness. Their friend was passing.

"I am so worried," one young woman messaged me with tight desperation in her words. "I know it's April's decision, but she is dying before she got right with God. She's chosen a different religion, and she will suffer the consequences. I feel so helpless because there's nothing I can do about it." Many felt helpless, unable to make April well.

Christians pray. It is our

opportunity to communicate with God. We pray before meals, when we rise in the morning, and when we go to bed at night. We pray when we covet the closeness of God, like a child who runs to their father when they're hurt or in need. We especially go to Him when someone is sick or dying.

I don't know how those of other faiths speak to their gods. I haven't studied the details of other religions, and haven't talked to April about it. Universities offer courses in comparative religions; however, I don't know if those syllabi include the gods in which April believes.

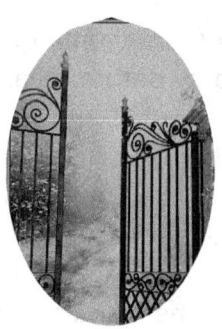

Thirteen

The Process

Praying someone to Heaven is a very special process. Set aside time for your "April," your family member, or friend. You will lead your loved one to the gate of Heaven.

I'm not saying that we save anyone. We have redemption through what Jesus did for us, not because of anything we could ever do on our own. My experience of guiding April along her path, was like the lamplighter, who trims his lamp, their lower light, to make sure the pathway home is well lit.

At Heaven's gate, speak their name onto the golden streets and marbled walls, so the melody of their name will sing along the flower-covered hills, and echo across the lush, green valleys. The majesty and beauty of this experience lack the proper words to express.

The Bible gives examples of prayers that changed other's lives. We read of Paul and Silas's time in jail. We learned that, when we accept salvation through Jesus Christ, we can name the members of our household and lead them to Christ, so they too can receive baptism.

It is not up to me to decide when it's too late for someone to meet the Lord. That is a decision only God will make. I am only to speak their name at the gate and introduce them to Heaven.

I followed the steps God gave me and felt at peace. I don't need to know the details. I believe that God is. I don't have to read His mind. That would not be a task I would hope to attempt – praise be to God. Speaking April's name into Heaven, it will reverberate there forever.

As I said, April is not a Christian. She'll take up that conversation when she gets home. It simply fell on my heart to pray her there. I followed this prompting from God, and what a holy experience it was.

These then are the steps given to my heart and understanding, to guide someone home. They can provide a template for you, too.

1. In prayer time, in the warm presence of God, see your loved one.
2. Call to them, using their name. Your family member or friend will hear you.
3. Tell them to walk with you as you lead them to the gate of Heaven and announce their presence within the garden.
4. Like the jailer told Paul, claim them as your family.
5. Bear witness on your loved one's behalf before the throne of God, claiming His blessings for them.
6. Ask God to cover them with His love, and welcome them home, through Christ Jesus.

From time to time over the next few days while they are still alive, call out their name, and directed them toward the gates of Heaven. Repeat this prayer often, and again once they pass. It is your belief in Jesus that makes this prayer possible.

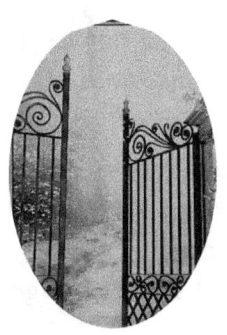

Fourteen

Pray Them to Heaven

Let me tell you how I experienced the blessing God gave me regarding April's homegoing. That Sunday morning, December 13, while April lay in a coma, the prayer came to me as an experience. I was both in it and observing it. I wrote the process down on my worship bulletin as fast as I could. Like a fleeting mist, the image was there and gone as soon as it passed. I prayed her to Heaven many times that day and beyond, using the outline I described.

I saw April walking through a haze, like a fog rising off the ocean in the morning when the light is just beginning to shine through.

With no doubt, I knew that my prayer put me in God's presence. I could feel Him there.

"April." When I called her name, she looked at me and smiled.

"Come with me." April fell in step beside me and together we walked to the beautiful, open gate of Heaven.

Into the garden beyond, I announced, "April is here. April is part of my family. I claim her. She's my daughter-in-law. Please cover her with your love, and welcome her home through the name of my savior,

Christ Jesus."

I bore witness on her behalf. "April loves and cares for our son, Vonn, and their children."

Then I prayed, "Father, God, you created the entire world with your words of love. I ask that your kingdom include April, that she may do your will in Heaven. I am here to bear witness on April's behalf. She is part of my family and is a good wife and mother. Loving people love her in return. She doesn't know you, Father, but I know her, and I believe you are God of all. I ask that Christ, your son, redeem her and that you cover her with your love, and welcome her into Paradise. Forgive me if I didn't speak to her enough on your behalf. Father, you are all glorious, loving, and forgiving. In the name of your son Jesus, my savior I pray. Amen."

• • •

December 14

April died December 14, 2020, at 2:40 AM. She is now in the arms of God.

It was my joy to light the way, to direct April to the gate, to speak her name, and to claim her as a member of my family. I cannot imagine that anyone, who would finally stand at the gate to Glory, would decide not to enter. Think of the amazing beauty, the melodic harmonies of the music, and the loved ones who went before, all gathered around, celebrating her homecoming. What a glorious day.

You ask, "What If my loved one died before I read this book, and called out their name?"

They are still reachable. Their living soul is somewhere. Call to them – they can hear you – lead them to the gate.

You may argue, "That is not my

experience."

No, it is mine, and I share it with you. Pray them to Heaven. Someday, you too will enjoy your homecoming. There will be a great celebration in Heaven, in praise to God, just because you came home.

REFERENCES

Eshraghi, Rebecca Sherry. April 13, 2020. Quantum Entanglement, Prayer, and Healing. Accessed 2/26/2021

https://bahaiteachings.org/quantum-entanglement-prayer-healing/ 2/26/2021.

Paredes, Adriana MA, Med, SAI Staff. Remote Healing Through Prayer. Spiritual Arts Institute. Accessed 2/15/2021 https://spiritualarts.org/blog/spiritual-healing/remote-healing-through-prayer/

Parker, William, Dr., and Elaine St. John (1962) *Prayer Can Change Your Life.* Prentice Hall

Rapp, Doris Gaines, Ph.D. (2014) *Prayer Therapy of Jesus.* Daniel's House Publishing.

Wikipedia. Wicca. Accessed 2/15/2021.
https://en.wikipedia.org/wiki/Wicca

About the Author

Doris Gaines Rapp, Ph.D. — Author, Psychologist, Catalyst

Dr. Rapp has written several non-fiction books. They often follow the needs of her clients, continuing education programs she leads, and/or programs that organizations ask her to give. Rather than re-inventing them each time, she collects the many hand-outs into a book.

As a psychologist, Rapp has directed the counseling centers at Taylor University, Upland, Indiana, and Bethel University, Mishawaka, Indiana. She has been an adjunct professor at St, Francis University in Fort Wayne, and Huntington University in Huntington, Indiana.

After moving nineteen times, Doris Gaines Rapp now writes full-time. Relocating frequently was hard. She now visits the people and places she loves in the characters and scenes within her many novels. She relives the experiences in her life through the images in her mind, then transfers those sights and sounds into words on paper.

As a psychologist for many years, she understands people, their motives, and dreams, and therefore can delve more deeply into the characters in her practice and novels. As a motivational speaker, she is a catalyst for individual change. Dr. Rapp recently received the Marquis Who's Who Lifetime Achievement Award.

She and her husband, Pastor Bill, hope to travel more when he retires … someday … for the fourth time.

Other Books by Doris Gaines Rapp

<u>*Novels*</u>:

Tucker McBride
Tucker McBride's Many Lives
Tucker McBride's Perfect Day
    (summer 2021)
Escape from the Belfry
Escape from the Shadows
Murder, She Blogged – Just in Time
News at Eleven – A Novel
Length of Days – The Age of Silence
(1st in the trilogy)
Length of Days – Beyond the Valley of the Keepers (2nd in the trilogy)
Length of Days – Search for Freedom
Hiawassee – Child of the Meadow
Smoke from Distant Fires

<u>Children's Picture Book:</u>
Shyloe and the Mayor
Lincoln's Christmas Mouse

Collection:
Christmas Feather, one of eight short stories by eight different authors in a collection titled, *Christmases Past*

Nonfiction:
Prayer Therapy of Jesus
Promote Yourself
Waiting for Jesus in a Can't Wait World – Advent 2014

Internet Presence

Facebook: Doris Gaines Rapp – Author Page

www.tuckermcbrideintheclassroom.com
https://prayertherapyofjesus.blogspot.com

www.dorisgainesrapp.comhttps://praythemtoheaven.blogspot.net

www.dorisgainesrapp.blogspot.com

dorisgainesrapp@gmail.com

https://.prayertherapyrapp.blogspot.com (old)

www.ingramcontent.com/pod-product-compliance
Lightning Source LLC
Chambersburg PA
CBHW072204100526
44589CB00015B/2353